CONTENTS

SECTION 1: WHY YOU ARE SPENDING HOURS AT THE GYM AND NOT SEEING RESULTS

CHAPTER 1: HOW THIS BOOK WILL HELP YOU

Kickboxing class. Jogging for miles. Spinning. Lifting light weights for 'toning'.

Do any of these activities sound familiar to you? Have these activities failed you??

You're in luck. Welcome to the book that's going to change the way you think about exercise and finally help you get the body you have always wanted.

For many of you, daily works outs are a way of life. Your day isn't complete if you don't get that sweat session in! Whether you sneak out of bed at the crack of dawn to hit the elliptical or you force yourself to make a stop on the way home from a 10-hour day at your job to ensure you burn those 400 calories, cardio gets done. The more cardio you do, the more calories you burn, right?

It's pretty nuts that you've been able to keep this schedule up for as long as you have! Furthermore, take a closer look at yourself. What's changed? Are you looking leaner? Are you looking slimmer? More toned? Do you feel *good*?

Chances are that the only thing you've accomplished is becoming a cardio professional. You aren't looking much better than when you first started despite the fact that you've spent more hours at the gym than some professional athletes have spent training for their career.

Others of you have realized that weight lifting is important, and have started weight lifting classes at the gym. Or maybe you have started lifting those 10 lb weights for countless reps. Other days you do a circuit with the machines. You make sure to get a 'weight lifting' session in every day in order to tone. But you're still flabby!

So who is this book for? And why should you read it??

This book is for women like you who aren't new to working out, but are fed up with the results they're getting. Motivation isn't necessarily your issue, but frustration is slowly taking over. You need a plan that actually works. You look ok in clothes, but with all the hours you spend busting ass in the gym you deserve to look good naked! You may have been a regular gym-goer for the last ten years, or maybe it's been just six long months with minimal results. Either way, you're sick of it! And, more importantly, you're ready for a change. The definition of insanity is doing the same thing over and over again and expecting different results. You know if you continue on the path you're on now, you will be looking at yourself in another six months seeing the same reflection in the mirror. Only now, you've wasted more time in your life chasing a seemingly unattainable goal. That sucks!

This book is for women who are ready to let go of their old training methods and cardio obsession and step forward into a realm where fat loss and looking hot is achieved without cardio.

Yes, you read that right. *Weight loss and looking great is achieved* <u>*without cardio*</u>.

If you can relate to this, then get ready because what you're going to learn is going to destroy all your previous perceptions of fat loss and excite the hell out of you.

CHAPTER 2: WHO AM I AND WHY SHOULD YOU LISTEN TO ME?

By now you might be wondering just who I am and why you should be listening to me. I will begin by telling you who I am not.

I am not a trainer or fitness model who gets paid to work out. I am also not someone who has made a career of writing about fitness. And finally, I am not someone who is blessed with good genetics.

Quite simply, I'm someone who has been there, done that. Name a diet – I did it. Name a workout, I tried it. Just like the hundreds of other exercise books I've devoured hoping that there would be one that finally broke me free from my, what I used to call, 'bad genes'.

Only it wasn't bad genes, it was stupidity. Not necessarily on my end – I thought I was doing everything right. The problem was that I was searching and learning from all the wrong sources. Lucky for you, the right source is right in front of your eyes. This book is a compilation of all the information from dozens of fitness experts whose programs I have read through and experimented with over the years. The fact that you are reading this book signals that you are at the end of your journey to find the secret to losing fat in the most effective and efficient way.

The weight loss battle ground is a hard place to be. Everywhere you turn, someone is throwing a different opinion at you! Eat low carb, eat Paleo, go vegan. Who do you listen to??

Others say that the new Pilates class they're doing is the greatest thing since sliced bread. So you try it, and it does nothing. If anything, it just dehydrated you, made you look like a human pretzel, and had you flapping your arms like you were preparing for lift-off.

I've even had dozens of 'professional' opinions from trainers that I thought could help me, but still, no progress. True, I may have been in the best cardiovascular shape of my life from all those hours and hours on the cardio machines. But, I felt like shit.

Almost any daily activity would tire me out quickly because my body was exhausted from all my hard work at spinning class earlier in the day. I had no energy after I got home for the evening and only wanted to hit the couch – if I could make it that far, that is.

On the weekends I'd forge on though, often going for two hour or longer bike rides while chasing after my dream to drop a few pounds.

Despite all this physical activity, my pants never became looser. I was buying the same size clothes that I had previously bought years ago and in some weeks even those started to feel tight.

My 'weight training' sessions were not working either. I still looked soft and flabby no matter how many reps I did.

I must mention that throughout this whole time I was trying to eat well. Sure, I may have tried the odd fad diet approach here and there but for the most part I made sure what I was putting in my body wasn't greasy, fatty, or high carb.

Just like you are right now, I was so frustrated at the way I was feeling and the results that I was seeing that I just wanted to throw in the towel. Maybe I would never get skinny? Perhaps it was just in my genes to be a little thick – either that, or my metabolism was just in an all out war against me.

I often wondered how so many women out there maintained such a svelte figure while I struggled so much. What was I missing? What did they know that I did not? They didn't seem to spend hours on the cardio machines doing their time! I hardly ever saw a woman with my 'dream' body in the gym next to me on the bike. So what was going on?

It wasn't until I got totally fed up and quit the cardio and the 'toning' routine that I really realized what was going on. Now, I want to share this secret with you.

I'm no expert trainer, I'm just a woman like you who has been subjected to so much information about weight loss and different theories that I was confused.

It's overwhelming at times, trying to weed through everything and figure out right from wrong. Some women get so lost up in the information search that they don't even *get* to the program at all. These women are the lucky ones, however, since they don't end up wasting hours of their life chained to those cardio machines and pink weights.

That's why I decided to write this book. I don't want you to go through what I went through. I want to see you succeed. Since I've finally started seeing success with my own training, it pains me to see the chick next to me making the exact same mistakes I did.

Sometimes I even try to explain to a woman I see in the gym what she's doing wrong. But often, she's so stuck in her ways that she fails to consider other possibilities. "There's sweat dripping down my head, so my workout it working!" "If I lift light weights, I'll get toned and not look like a man!" Open your mind. It's the only way you will make any progress. It comes down to using the right methods and changing the way you think.

If you're not ready to change your thinking and leave behind your former beliefs, you're going to be held back. Stuck in a world where each day begins with a cardio session and ends with 100 situps.

If you have the tenacity to break free from that world, then by following the advice I'm going to share with you, you can. I GUARANTEE you that if you follow the method given in this book, you WILL lose fat. I'm not saying it's simple and you'll get results instantly. If there was a magic wand I could wave that would make you ten pounds lighter, believe me I'd do that (well actually, I'd probably patent it first and make a few million), but there isn't.

True fat loss – fat loss that sticks with you and doesn't return a month after you come off your diet is the result of hard work. But this hard work is also smart work, so you'll require less of it to see results.

And trust me, it doesn't take many changes to make it 'less work' than what you're likely doing right now. As any cardio-addicted chick knows, the gym could very easily be termed her home away from home.

Before we dive into the methods that I'm going to share with you, let's have a brief discussion about the typical approach to weight loss most women follow. Then you'll be able to compare this to what I'm going to share with you and you'll see the differences that are involved.

CHAPTER 3: THE AVERAGE WOMAN'S APPROACH TO WEIGHT LOSS – WHERE DID WE GO WRONG

For most women, the main focus when they get themselves on a weight loss program is on two things: diet and cardio training. Light 'toning' exercises may be included as well. After all, as the saying goes, 'to lose weight, eat less and move more'. Boy do some women take that to heart – my former self included.

The problem is not that these women are not dedicated to sticking with their plan (because many do just that with Nazi-like determination), but instead that their plan sucks to begin with.

The typical workout schedule for most women includes at least two solo cardio sessions spent on their choice of machine (the bike, the treadmill, or the elliptical), two more group cardio exercises sessions (kick-boxing spin class, or some other form), as well as possibly some type of stretching or yoga in effort to mix it up. Cardio is followed up by some "toning" exercises, such as the butt blaster or some other machine.

In some cases, she may go back into the gym later on in the day and perform a second session as well, depending on how much she feels it's going to help her lose the weight and whether time permits.

These women often feel very weighed down by their obligation to get that cardio in. In some instances, they may even withhold food until the cardio has been performed. The thinking here is 'I can eat it if I burn it off first'. In other instances, they feel like they can make up for eating too much by doing cardio. After all, 'I can just burn off the calories I ate'.

Both cases are not conducive to losing fat. Let's go through a couple of examples:

If you ask the first kind of average woman (we'll call her "eat-like-a-bird Brittany") to tell you about her diet it might go something like this:

Morning: Wake up and have a cup of coffee with a piece of fruit, and maybe a small low-fat yogurt. Yummy.

Mid-morning: Starving! More coffee – have to push through until lunch.

Lunch: Large lettuce salad with cherry tomatoes and half a can of tuna. One small cookie. Wishing for 5 more cookies.

Mid-Afternoon: A small bag of carrots along with a 100 calorie snack sized bar. So tired. Still starving.

Dinner: A small plate of pasta with at least two cups of cooked vegetables and a very small piece of chicken or fish.

Before bed: Tea – eating before bed makes you gain weight, right?

The other kind of average women is one who likes the idea of not eating a lot of calories throughout the day, but in reality only makes it until dinnertime. Let's refer to her as "night-binge Nancy". Her diet goes something like this.

Morning: Wake up and have a cup of coffee with egg whites and grapefruit. So healthy! Nancy feels skinny.

Mid-morning: Almonds and 4 pieces of sugar free gum. Almost lunch time. Doing good.

Lunch: Half a small chicken sandwich on wheat bread, dry. Somewhat satisfied!

Mid-Afternoon: Not needed, Nancy is making it until dinner!

Dinner: Nancy met a new boy who invited her out to dinner and drinks at a fabulous Italian restaurant. She vowed to eat light. After 2 "carbless" vodka-sodas, Nancy is starving, happy, and no longer cares about her diet. She eats all the bread on the table, a large fettuccini alfredo, and finishes off with a large piece of Tiramisu.

The Next Morning: Nancy wakes up feeling fat, hating life, and does two hours of hung-over cardio followed by 500 crunches on the ab machine.

If you are anything like Brittany or Nancy, you could definitely be summarized as the average dieting woman. Both of these diets lack nutrients, calories, and most importantly, protein. While each of these diets are different, both have there own set of problems.

By the time you pair this dietary strategy together with all the loads of cardio that's being done on the workout side of things, you have yourself a major problem.

Another big issue that often surfaces with the average woman on a weight loss program is diet pills. It doesn't take much to figure out just how many different variations of diet pills there are available right now – just run a quick search through the Internet or walk through any supplement store in the 'Weight Loss' section.

Each diet pill has its own claim to fame but one commonality among them all is the promise of rapid, easy weight loss.

Think about this though: If weight loss really could be 'rapid and easy', don't you think doctors would be handing out these pills and we'd just be done with the obesity problem altogether? "Lose 10 lbs in 10 days, no exercise!" Really? Let me ask you something, have you ever met anyone in your life who took diet pills, lost weight, and lived happily ever after in their skinny and healthy life?

Just like those idiots who hunt down get-rich-quick schemes only to find themselves broke as a kid in a candy shop a few months later when their plan fails, you'll find the same with weight loss. If you're going to rely on quick weight loss plans or pills, you're going to find that you may lose some quick weight, but just as quickly that weight will come right back on. More often than not, you will gain back more than you lost.

This doesn't even take into account the fact that often these weight pills can impose health risks on some individuals since they contain stimulatory properties that can speed up your heart rate, mess with your concentration levels, and cause your body to feel very jittery and nervous, especially if you're already sensitive to substances like caffeine. You will look skinny, hot, and cracked out!

Diet pills do quite well in the market though because of all these female dieters just like Brittany and Nancy who are on programs that aren't delivering results and want a change. Rather than looking at the source of their problem – that program they are on, they look for an outside factor that will help them beat the weight loss game.

I know this because I was one of those people. I searched for my 'quick-fix' by jumping from workout plan to workout plan and diet to diet. I tried a few different supplements thinking it would help boost my results, but they didn't. All they did was eat up money that could have been put to much better use.

We are so misinformed as a society, especially as women, about what works and what doesn't. We are the primary targets for weight loss products. Women seem to fear certain types of physical activity because all the big scary men are the ones in the weight room working on their big muscles. We are instead the ones who are in the cardio or the pink weight section of the gym working on getting trim

Sadly, rolling with the boys at the gym is what gets you results.

CHAPTER 4: THE CARDIO KILLER

Now that we've identified what the average woman's approach to weight loss looks like, it's time to identify why this is a huge problem. There are so many things wrong with this workout program, and there are so many ways you could make it better that it's hard to know where to start.

Some exercise is always better than no exercise, but there definitely comes a point where too much exercise is counterproductive. For the vast majority of women, 'too much cardio' is the single best statement to describe their workout approach.

<u>The Impacts Cardio Exercise Has On The Body</u>

It's important that you come to realize what the impact all this cardio activity on the body is so you can clearly see why you should stay way from it. If you look at two groups of athletes - marathon runners vs sprinters - you can clearly see the difference in body types.

Marathon runners tend to be very thin and almost gaunt looking, really lacking any form of muscle tone and definition. Sprinters, on the other hand, tend to be more muscular while still maintaining a feminine physique. They have a nice curvier shape to them and exude an image of strength. Both Britanny and Nancy want to look like the sprinter. Who do you want to look like?

In other cases, some marathon runners (the recreational variety that definitely are training hard but aren't running world class marathons) may actually appear slightly overweight. They're not fat by any means, but if you look closely they still lack that muscle definition. They're thin but have a sort of 'softness' to them. This softness can be described as skinny-fat.

Humans are creatures of habit by nature. As a result, the human body is very good at adapting to activities that are done over and over. When you're doing very high volumes of cardio training as with both recreational and professional marathon runners, the body is going to get tricked into thinking that it has to transport itself over long distances. Because of this, it's going to attempt to get rid of the heaviest, most costly tissue that it has first.

What type of tissue is this?

If you said muscle tissue, you're right! When doing cardio for extended periods of time, your body is going to catch on to the fact that the lighter it is, the better it will do. Since the same volume muscle is over twice as heavy as fat, your body chooses to get rid of muscle mass first. In addition, muscle mass requires way more energy to maintain itself on a daily basis compared to fat mass, so from a survival viewpoint, the less muscle mass you have, the better.

In order to conserve fuel used to perform those cardio workouts each day, your body must limit the amount of fuel it burns every minute. The best way to do this is to conserve the body fat (which conveniently also is the body's storage form of fuel) and get rid of the tissue that's too costly – muscle mass.

So what you have at the end of this cycle is a loss of lean muscle mass and the preservation of body fat. THAT'S why those marathoners look the way they do! Not exactly what you were hoping for in terms of body composition changes, was it?

To add to this problem, this change will only intensify the cycle. As you see yourself looking softer and softer you may decide to begin adding more and more cardio, burning up more of that precious muscle mass that used to help you have a high metabolic rate. Or you may decide to lift light weights for longer.

After months have passed you're now finding that you can hardly maintain your body weight on half the food you used to eat and in most cases, you're actually starting to *gain* more body fat.

At this stage in the game, you've just trained your body to start storing body fat. It has adapted quickly to all the demands being placed on it with all that cardio and it's reacting. Store body fat, burn off muscle. As for lifting the light weights, it simply does nothing.

Ladies, this is the hamster wheel at it's best. No matter how fast you run you will get NO WHERE. This is NOT the situation you want to be in.

Another big reason why so many women fall into this cardio trap is because they've heard so much about how you have to be in that 'fat burning zone' in order to see real fat loss. What this belief essentially states is that because your body utilizes fat as fuel when you work out at a lower intensity, and glucose as fuel when you workout at a higher intensity, you should perform the lower intensity forms of exercise instead.

Since most women are trying to burn off body fat, it would seem to only make sense to perform exercise that burns fat. Right?

Wrong! What you must remember with this is that fat loss doesn't come down to whether you're burning body fat calories or glucose calories. What it comes down to is if you burn off more than you took in at the end of the day.

If you've eaten more than you've burned off throughout the day, you won't lose weight. Likewise, if you burn off more calories than you take in, you're on the road to burning fat, regardless of when and how these calories are burned off.

Again, if you've consumed more than you've burned off, you

aren't going to be losing any body fat! So going back to that 'fat burning zone' myth - despite the fact that you may be using fat as fuel during this type of exercise, if you're hardly burning any calories at all there's a good chance that at the end of the day you will have still consumed more than you've burned off. Trust me, you don't have to be on Nancy's dinner date to consume more calories than you will burn off with these long, drawn out 'fat burning zone' workouts.

Let's look at an example to illustrate this.

Say you have two women who each burn 1400 calories just existing (no exercise, we are talking just to stay alive).

Now, one woman (Fat-Burning Zone Fern) goes and does her low intensity 'fat burning zone' cardio and burns off a whole 200 calories. Big deal.

So now, Fern burned 1600 calories over the course of that day.

Woman two (Smart Susan) goes and does an intense workout session that combines some aerobic based training with a number of heavy resistance exercises to really firm up her muscles. She burns 500 calories in that session.

Her total daily calorie burn now is 1900 calories.

Who loses more body fat?

If you said Smart Susan, you're starting to get the hang of this! It doesn't matter that Fern used fat as a fuel source during her workout while Susan used glucose (since high intensity exercise can only use glucose for fuel), all that matters is who burned more calories at the end of that day.

So hopefully now you can see why that fat burning zone is leading you astray. Sure, you may be burning fat as fuel, but that doesn't always mean you're *losing fat.* There's a big difference here – a difference it took me many years to learn, so I hope you can understand it much faster.

Finally, the last big problem with all that cardio training is the risk of injury. You've invested in that nice pair of running shoes and have become a serious runner! If you're out there pounding the pavement for hours each week, your chances of becoming injured are going to be pretty high. Whether it's a stress fracture, a pulled muscle, or you just not recovering properly between workouts, you're highly likely to find yourself injured sooner or later.

Without adequate rest in a weekly workout schedule, you'll never be able to recover and get stronger. Instead, you'll just grow weaker over time. Even professional athletes understand the importance of enough rest and schedule full days off into their program.

Not your average woman who wants weight loss, though! She's in there every single day of the week, never missing a beat. The amount of wear and tear this causes on the body is really quite extensive! For some women who have been doing way too much cardio for years it can take months before they're fully recovered after taking time off.

What's more is that very often all this exercise actually will make you *appear* larger as well, even though it's not actual fat gain. With all that exercise the body starts to become very inflamed, which causes it to store excess water in the tissues.

Some people actually find that after taking a week or so off cardio entirely, they look leaner than they ever did before. Muscle definition may even start to show now that all this inflammation has gone down. It's really quite the phenomenal occurrence, but one that many women never get the chance to see because they're married to the elliptical machine!

I should note that this effect is usually more predominant in the leg muscles since these are the ones that are utilized most during cardio training. So if you find that you're really lacking any leg muscle definition whatsoever, this could be what's happening to you.

If you can break from your cardio craziness, you may just find that you're looking better than ever.

Now you have a much better idea of all the problems associated with large volumes of cardio training. Sure, you will always have those people out there who get a physical high from long endurance workouts (often called the 'runners high') who wouldn't give that up to save their life.

But these women are not typically concerned with how they look. Their main goal is to get that "high" feeling from their workouts. They love endurance exercise, plain and simple. Call them what you want (we'll refer to them as Crazy), but that's not the target of this book.

The target audience of this book, and hopefully what describes you, is someone who *doesn't* love cardio exercise and quite matter-of-factly would love to get skinny without it. But, you're still scared to abandon your old cardio ways because you think without it you'll get fat.

That's the problem I'm trying to solve – to show you that there is another way, a far more effective way.

Before I dive into telling you about these methods, let's first take a short quiz to ensure that you are in fact suffering from the 'cardio overload' syndrome.

CHAPTER 5: ARE YOU A SLAVE TO THE WHEEL?

I n the following quiz I'm going to ask you a series of questions that should help assess just how bad your situation is. It's important to be brutally honest here with your answers because it's really going to reveal the truth – and that is what you want to know, right?

No one else is going to see these answers except yourself so there's no point in trying to pass it off as something it's not. Be open and honest. Assess your real situation so you know exactly where you stand on the spectrum.

Keep track of your answers as you go along and at the end I'll summarize where you are.

1. On average, you're doing cardio this many times per week:

a. Ten – yes, I'm aware there are not ten days in the week; I do multiple sessions on some days
b. Seven – once a day keeps the doctor away!
c. Five – I force myself to take weekends off, but often go on some type of walk, run, or cycle outdoors over the weekend
d. Three or four – I'd like to do more but my schedule just does not allow it

2. On average, how long do those cardio sessions last?

a. One hour – I like to get my calorie burn up to at least 500 calories per session
b. 45 minutes – I want to build up my endurance but can't stay in the gym for much more than this
c. 30 minutes – but I sometimes go back for a second round in the evening
d. 30 minutes or less – I get bored easily

3. When do you find yourself doing these workouts?

a. Morning, afternoon, evening – I'm in the gym so much I might as well sleep there
b. Morning – I want to get it over and done with before I start my day – otherwise, I may miss it
c. Right after work – I build it into my daily schedule
d. It varies depending on what I have going on

4. Before you do the workout, what's your diet like?

a. Diet? Are you crazy? Eating food is for losers.
b. Coffee – I need the caffeine to get me going. I might have a piece of fruit as well.
c. A mixed meal of carbohydrates and protein, which I typically eat at least an hour before
d. It varies based on where I am and if I have food with me.

5. Your primary cardio goal and the reason for doing cardio is:

a. To get skinny – but it's not working as I had expected it to
b. To lose weight but also maintain my health, that's important
c. To train for some type of endurance event and lose weight in the process
d. Because I want to go to the gym and don't know what else to do – this seems simple enough

<u>Your Assessment</u>

Take a look at your answers and see which letter was most predominant for you.

<u>Mostly A's</u>

If you answered mostly A's, you're in dire need of a workout make-over. Of all people, you're the one who's most hooked on your cardio habits and likely will have the hardest time trying to break free. The good news is that it is definitely possible if you really put your mind to it. As an added benefit, because of how improper the techniques you're using right now really are, you're going to see the greatest results by changing your ways.

Congratulations, you've earned yourself the title of a 'cardio queen'!

<u>Mostly B's</u>

If you found yourself answering mostly B's, you're right there along with the A person, however the situation is not quite as bad. You aren't so obsessed with getting in your cardio to lose weight that you'll skip all other things to get it done. You are also likely have a bit more balance in your life and aren't as fatigued on a regular basis from the cardio you're doing.

Still, you definitely have some major changes to make if you want to see good results.

<u>Mostly C's</u> If you answered mostly C, you are definitely hooked on cardio, but you're teetering on the edge of being able to easily switch over and adopt new habits. You're probably someone who hasn't been playing the cardio game all that long and still hasn't realized that you aren't going to see the results you're looking for.

You may not be all that frustrated yet because you honestly don't feel as though it's taking over your life. You get it in regularly but it's not something that has to be done – like breathing. It's there because you think it will help you lose weight. If you keep going at this pace however, you could become an A or B person.

<u>Mostly D's</u>

If you find you fall into this category, the great news is that you aren't all that stuck in your ways yet. It's going to be a fairly easy change for you to move over to a more effective program. You're doing the cardio because you aren't really sure what else you can do although you want to do SOMETHING.

Good.

You have that motivation to get in better shape and look great, you just need more information in general about exercise training. You're in the best position of everyone to really take the information you learn here and put it to use immediately.

You likely won't have any of those cardio 'mind demons' that are telling you otherwise because you aren't chained to your favorite piece of cardio equipment like the A woman is.

So where do you stand after taking this quiz? Note that no matter where you're at, change is possible, but you have to be willing to work at it. For many women stuck in the cardio game, the mental aspect of leaving it behind is far greater than any of the physical challenges they'll face with the new exercise routine.

Often, this fear is the hardest thing to overcome because it involves training the mind to think a new way, and this new way is often led with a bit of fear. Right now you probably feel like your daily cardio session is the only thing that's keeping you from packing on the pounds.

I hope you really do give it an honest shot and listen to the advice I'm about to give you because it will make such a big difference in your life. Not only will you feel better and have more energy each day, but you're going to look better as well. And that's not to mention the fact that you'll have freed up at least an hour a day to do other things that you can enjoy.

Who doesn't need an extra hour in the day?

So let's get started and show you how you can leave this destructive workout pattern behind and get yourself on a new and improved path that's going to change your life forever.

CHAPTER 6: BREAK FREE – AND GET RESULTS

Right now, you are under the impression that you must work hard – and long to get good results in the gym. It's not uncommon for you to put in upwards of six to seven hours a week exercising. For some this can even jump up to twenty hours or more, all depending on how fat you feel that particular week.

You are going to be totally surprised when you realize just how little time it really takes to see the results that you are after. If you're doing the right types of exercise, a complete body transformation can take place in as little as thirty minutes, three times a week.

You read that right. You do not need to make the gym your home-away-from-home. The key is to work smarter, not harder. What I am going to teach and show you throughout this book is how you can tailor your workouts so that after you perform them, you continue to burn more calories for the rest of the day.

That means later on in the evening when you're being lazy on the couch, your metabolism is burning up calories faster than ever before.

Stop and think about this for a second. How many hours, right now, do you spend in the gym? One? Maybe two? And how many hours are there in the day? Since there are twenty-two to twenty-three hours that you are not in the gym, wouldn't it make sense that if you could maximize how many calories you were burning during this time you would see far superior progress? Even if you could burn 10% more calories each hour of the day than what you did before, that would easily translate into almost 200 calories over the course of the day.

200 calories per day at thirty days per month would mean almost two additional pounds of fat off your body each month. Vanished – with no effort whatsoever on your part!

If you can rev up that metabolic rate using all the techniques I'm going to show you, progress will come automatically. The big problem is that right now you're using all the techniques which actually just slow the body down, so instead of seeing some serious movement forward with your goals, you are actually starting to move backward – or staying stagnant.

The Weight Loss Pyramid

Now, you have likely heard about the food pyramid before (which shouldn't exactly be followed, but we'll get to more on that issue in a minute), but what you probably haven't had the chance to see is the weight loss pyramid.

What this pyramid essentially represents is the different aspects of weight loss and how they must be integrated into your overall plan. Just like the food pyramid, certain aspects take up a much greater portion of importance, while others are much closer to the top.

The Bottom Of The Pyramid

At the bottom of the pyramid lies your diet. This section should take up approximately 75% of the total pyramid because diet is that important when it comes to getting results. Keep in mind, however, that I'm not talking about a very low calorie diets that hardly provide you any sustenance.

I'm talking about diets that supply you with all the essential nutrients that you need to see the best results from your program while still getting your body to use fat for fuel. When you eat properly, you'll actually be able to eat way more calories than you previously thought while still being able to lose weight.

Diet will make or break fat loss results!

For example, how many calories are you burning on your average cardio workout? 300? 500, if you're really putting in time?

And how many calories are in a piece of gourmet cheesecake? 600? 800 perhaps? Each chocolate chip cookie you eat has about 150 calories, so eat a few and you are at 500 calories easily! As you can see, those five minutes spent indulging in that cheesecake or cookies can easily wipe out an hour or more on the cardio machines, proving both that cardio is ineffective for overall fat loss and that you should never attempt to try and compensate for a bad diet with exercise.

If diet tends to be a big hurdle for you, then you have lots of work to do. However, with the diet tricks I'm going to discuss you will likely find that creating a fat loss plan that delivers is not nearly as difficult as it may seem.

The Middle Of The Pyramid

Next we come to the middle of the pyramid. This is where your resistance training lies. When it comes to THE exercise to perform to drop body fat and entirely reshape your body, this is the one that's going to get you results.

So out of our entire pyramid, resistance exercise comprises about 20% of all results. Remember that when we are referring to results we are strictly talking about fat loss. In an overall health outlook as well as weight maintenance outlook, resistance training is a very important factor. It may even possibly take up 40% while diet moves closer to 50% or so.

This is due to the fact that long-term resistance training will really help boost your lean body tissue, revving your metabolic rate and making it easier to eat more calories while staying lean. What does this mean? If you lift weights you can actually burn fat while sitting on your ass!

The Top Of The Pyramid

At the top of the pyramid, making up 5% or less, is cardio training. I'm not even talking about scheduled cardio– that can be completely eliminated from the pyramid as far as I'm concerned.

This portion of the pyramid comprises all the exercise you do in your daily life – walking to the store, mowing the grass, cleaning the house, and so on. All can be considered cardiovascular because it gets you moving and keeps your heart at a slightly elevated pace. These activities burn calories and - though not significantly - over time these calories can add up.

This portion of the pyramid does contribute a small amount to your weight loss program, which is why it's rated up there at the very top.

So, how does this pyramid compare to the one you are currently following? What does your personal pyramid look like? Is cardio on the bottom of the pyramid for you? If so, then you have some serious changes to make.

It's important that you really do make the commitment to try and change your ways if you want to break free from this weight loss game once and for all. Don't think that you can just add in what I'm going to tell you and keep up with those cardio workouts 'just in case'. This won't work. Your body will end up vastly over-trained, incredibly fatigued, and become a breeding ground for weight gain.

Now, let's go over your new solution.

CHAPTER 7: YOUR RESISTANCE TRAINING SOLUTION

If you're ready to make some major changes in how you look, resistance training is the solution for you. Resistance training definition: Any form of exercise where your muscles work against a high-intensity stimulus that only lasts for a brief period of time. This does NOT count cardio that's performed at a higher level (such as biking at level 10).

We're talking exercise that lasts just twenty to forty seconds at a time. This all-out burst is going to spark your metabolic rate and get you to burn calories faster than you ever have in the past. Also, since you're adding in intensity, you're going to notice your muscles taking on a nicer shape and becoming more lean and defined. Rather than that soft, 'jiggle-like' appearance they may have had, your muscles will now be firm and toned.

Resistance training can come in many forms: free weights, weight machines, resistance bands, TRX, Ultimate Sandbag, etc. You definitely have your pick of options to do this exercise with.

What is important to note is that you really must *challenge* yourself. I'm not talking about going to the gym and picking up those pink weights and doing a few curls or doing the machines.

How many times have you gone into the gym and headed straight for the nautilus machine? You may have been thinking you were doing the right thing, but ask yourself when the last time was that you saw a change in your body?

Rather than using those machines for your resistance workouts, you need to step it up and move into the free weights section. This is the best place to stimulate your muscle fibers to the fullest extent while working the core at the same time.

If you want a lean mid-section, free weights is where it's at!

Be sure that you're lifting *heavy*. Don't go for something light that you can lift twenty times. Aim for a weight that really is going to test your strength to the max.

Do not be scared to lift heavy weights – that's where progress is made!

I'm going to repeat this so it gets drilled into your mind since it's extremely important - *Do not be scared to lift heavy weights!*

If you think that you're going to get big and bulky if you so much as look at the weight room, I've got news for you - As a woman, you do not have nearly enough testosterone flowing through your body to ever really 'bulk' up.

Those women that you may see competing in bodybuilding competitions that do look quite manly are using some form of chemical enhancement (taking testosterone injections). I guarantee you.

Since you are definitely not going to do this, you don't have to worry. Women are not physiologically designed to get bulky.

Instead, what lifting the heavier weights will do is increase how many calories you burn every single minute of the day, increase your strength levels, and help you lose all that fat off your body that's hiding your muscle definition.

Doesn't that sound fantastic?

I thought so.

Say goodbye to light weights and start challenging yourself. Even if this means buying equipment and working out at home.

If the weight room scares you, work out in your living room. It's still no excuse *not* to get your heavy strength training in. One viable option you have to work out at home is by using the TRX Suspension Trainer system.

If you've never had a look at what this system is all about, now is definitely the time to do so. It's a rather simplistic rope system, but the results it generates can be quite phenomenal.

This system can be taken with you wherever you go and allows you to perform numerous different exercises which are going to really target every single muscle in your body. From your legs to your abs to your arms, you will not miss out on anything when using this system.

Also, don't think that you can just join one of those weight lifting classes at the gym and be done with it. Those aren't much better than a few random bicep curls with the pink weights and are not going to get you the results you're looking for.

Many of these classes are still very cardio based workouts and are just going to keep you in the same destructive pattern you've been on for so long. You need a quality resistance-training workout that's going to push your physical capabilities and produce results.

That is what I'm going to give you here.

So now that you understand the type of workout you'll be doing, let's go over a few of the different resistance training options. These include full body workouts, split body workouts, circuit training workouts, and boot camp workouts.

<u>Full Body Workouts</u>

The full body workout option is great for those of you who are looking for something that doesn't have as large of a time commitment since you'll only be required to be in the gym three days a week (or two if you're really pressed for time).

Full body workouts also tend to produce a very nice metabolic response since you're working so many muscle fibers all at once. When you begin splitting up the body you'll be working only certain groups of muscles at a time, so the overall calorie burn may be slightly lower (don't worry, you'll make up for it with more frequent gym visits).

Either way, full body workouts are very effective for getting excellent fat loss results and are good for those who are just getting started. They will allow you to focus on the main core exercises that will round out your program and the ones that help you see great progress right off the bat.

With the full body workout approach you won't be performing very many isolated exercises. Those aren't the major calorie-burners anyway though, so not that big of a deal.

<u>Upper/Lower Splits</u>

The second type of workout is the upper and lower body split. With this type of set-up you'll be going into the gym and working the upper body one day and lower body the next.

You will rest on the third day and then repeat the two day cycle again to round out the week. Weekends are taken off and are used for extra rest and recovery so you can be sure you're coming back to this workout stronger than ever before.

Since you are breaking the body up in half you can perform more exercises for each muscle group. Therefore, those who are looking for some really big changes will want to use this approach. For example, if you're looking to get toned shoulders in order to look great in sleeveless dresses, you can add a few extra shoulder exercises into your upper body day without the workout becoming incredibly long.

One thing that is important to always keep in the back of your mind is that you can't spot reduce through weight training. For example, if you want a six-pack, you aren't going to get it by doing hundreds of sit-ups each day. Similarly, if you have a lot of fat under your arms, don't expect tricep extensions to remove it.

In order to get the toned look, you have to remove the fat first. Then, if you're doing proper strength training exercises the muscle will become visible – resulting in what is popularly known as the 'toned' look.

<u>Circuit Training</u>

The third type of resistance program is circuit training. Circuit training DOES NOT mean using light weights and squeezing out as many reps as you can before moving to the next station. That type of approach is strikingly similar to the cardio workouts we're trying to get away from, and as I already mentioned, light weights are your enemy right now!

Just to be clear, workouts that require you to squeeze out maximum reps in an allotted interval do have a place in a fat loss program. This style is typically used in bootcamp workouts, which you will learn more about in the next section. These circuit workouts are NOT to be confused with a circuit that consists of moving through a series of machines.

The type of circuit training you should be focusing on now consists of performing a group of five or six key weight lifting exercises and moving between them quickly. You will be lifting a relatively heavy weight, meaning that you will fatigue by the twelfth rep. Nonetheless, immediately after that exercise is completed you're going to move to the next exercise as quickly as possible.

The reduced rest periods in this type of workout tend to boost the metabolism up even higher, so now you get the benefits of lifting heavier weights along with added fat burning.

Note that you will not lift as heavy of a weight as you would if you were using the longer rest periods since the recovery time is much shorter. However, that does NOT mean you should ease up to the point of being back at the pink weights. Challenge yourself!

Also, you should alternate upper body exercises with lower body exercises while progressing through your circuit training workout. This allows the upper body to rest while the lower body works, thereby increasing the chances that you can maintain that heavier weight.

Typically, circuit style training programs are performed using a full body approach since you have the upper/lower alternating pattern in there.

Ideally, you will perform three or four circuit training workouts a week, being sure to switch up the exercises you use with each session.

<u>Bootcamp Workouts</u>

Finally we come to the last type of resistance training workout - the bootcamp workout.

This workout has more of a cardiovascular component than your traditional strength training programs. However, it definitely still utilizes a variety of bodyweight exercises in order to help increase your muscular strength. The bodyweight exercises are key to producing the outcome you are going for with your workout.

In bootcamp, you will perform exercises such as push-ups, pull-ups, bodyweight squats, lunges, burpees, and so on.

If you choose to do bootcamp workouts, you should still get two full body strength based workouts in a week. The reason for this is that you still need to push against weight resistance since it taxes the body in a different way.

So there you have it! These are all the main workouts that should make up your week. After a few sessions of each one you will very likely be hooked for life and will never want to go back to your old, boring cardio sessions again.

CHAPTER 8: PUTTING TOGETHER YOUR PLAN FOR SUCCESS

Now we must get into the nitty-gritty details of what your workout is going to look like. The following is the specifics of what you should be doing each and every time you go into the gym. I'm going to present you with a full body workout program, an upper/lower split workout program, and a circuit training workout program.

We won't go into details of the bootcamp workout since each instructor will have their own preference for how they want to run this.

Always remember that just because you choose one workout type of start with, it does not mean you're stuck with it for the long term. It's always a good idea to change something over time since it keeps your body guessing. This 'unknown' ensures that you'll never hit a plateau.

If you want to keep seeing progress, be sure that you're constantly pushing your body past your comfort zone.

Full Body Workout Program

The following workouts are to be performed on a Monday, Wednesday, and Friday schedule. If that doesn't work for you, you could do Tuesday, Thursday, Saturday (or Sunday). Just make sure that you have at least one full day of rest between workouts. It's critical that you give each muscle group 48 hours to recover. One important thing to remember for all you type A's: if you miss one workout because you have a hot date, or because you just feel crappy that day - guess what will happen? NOTHING! If you miss a workout, no big deal, just go the next day. Life is never linear.

With the following exercises, you want to select a weight that will have you feeling pooped by the time you hit the last rep. You should be tired enough to feel like you can't perform another one without sacrificing your ability to maintain good form, but not so tired that you have to call it quits.

You're going to work across a few different rep ranges within this workout. Rep ranges of 5-8 reps are primarily geared towards helping you increase your strength level, while the 8-12 rep range is directed at increasing your metabolic rate (while still also helping you develop some muscular strength).

There's no need to go higher than 12 reps. If you can lift your weight more than this it means you aren't lifting as heavy of a weight as you theoretically could and will not see the type of re-sults that you're after.

You will gain strength quicker than you think! Every two work-outs or so you will need to add weight to feel challenged by the

12th rep. It should NEVER get easier.

Aim for about forty-five to sixty seconds of rest when you are working in the lower rep range (lifting a heavier weight will re-quire more rest time), and aim for thirty seconds of rest for the 8-12 rep exercises. The rest should be short and snappy. This is what will get that metabolism of yours really cranking!

Remember that you should start each workout with a short warm-up and cool-down. This means about 5 minutes of brisk walking or biking to get the blood moving. This should NOT be a full-fledged cardio session!

If you are unfamiliar with how to do any of the following exercises, please refer to a little website called YouTube. Put in the name of the exercise as the keyword in the search, and pick your choice of live demos.

Monday:

Exercise	Sets	Reps	Rest
Chest Press	4	6	60 seconds
Squats	4	6	60 seconds
Bent Over Barbell Rows	3	8	45 seconds
Deadlifts	4	6	45 seconds
Hanging Leg Raise	2	12	30 seconds

Wednesday:

Exercise	Sets	Reps	Rest
Incline Bench Press	3	8	45 seconds
Lunges	3	8	45 seconds
Lateral-Pull-Down	3	8	45 seconds
Step-Ups	3	8	45 seconds
Standing Calf Raises	2	12	30 seconds

Friday:

Exercise	Sets	Reps	Rest
Chest Press	4	6	60 seconds
Squats	4	6	60 seconds
Shoulder Press	3	8	45 seconds
Bent Over Barbell Rows	3	8	45 seconds
Deadlifts	3	8	45 seconds
Sit-Ups On An Exercise Ball	2	12	30 seconds

Upper/Lower Split Workout Program

Next we move on to the upper/lower body split. As stated above, this is a good option for those who are looking to specialize a bit more with their workout strategy. With each workout you will be able to add a few more exercises for a particular body part if needed.

Similar to the full body workout, you'll work across a variety of different rep ranges. Remember, lift heavy! Be sure not to 'save' yourself for later on in the workout by working with less than your maximum weight. It is ALWAYS better to have a shorter, more intense workout.

Push yourself! You're a lot stronger than you think if you just put forth that effort. If you find yourself too tired to continue, get out of the gym and make sure you're well rested for your next workout.

Again, YouTube comes in handy here.

Monday

Exercise	Sets	Reps	Rest
Bench Press	4	6	60 seconds
Bent Over Row	4	6	60 seconds
Shoulder Press	3	8	45 seconds
Upright Row	3	8	45 seconds
Bicep Curl	2	12	30 seconds
Tricep Extension	2	12	30 seconds
Lateral Raise	2	12	30 seconds

Tuesday

Exercise	Sets	Reps	Rest

Squats	4	6	60 seconds
Deadlifts	4	6	60 seconds
Leg Extension	3	8	45 seconds
Hamstring Curl	3	8	45 seconds
Standing Calf Raises	2	12	30 seconds
Hanging Leg Raises	2	12	30 seconds
Exercise Ball Sit-Ups	2	12	30 seconds

Wednesday: Rest

Thursday

Exercise	Sets	Reps	Rest
Incline Bench Press	3	8	45 seconds
Lateral Pull-Down	3	8	45 seconds
Chest Fly's	3	8	45 seconds
Reverse Fly's	3	8	45 seconds
Bicep Curls	2	12	30 seconds
Tricep Extensions	2	12	30 seconds
Front Raises	2	12	30 seconds

Friday

Exercise	Sets	Reps	Rest
Squats	3	8	45 seconds
Lunges	3	8	45 seconds
Leg Extensions	2	12	30 seconds
Hamstring Curls	2	12	30 seconds
Seated Calf Raises	2	12	30 seconds
Back Hyperextension	2	12	30 seconds

Lying Leg Raises	2	12	30 seconds

Saturday and Sunday: Rest

As you can see, your Monday /Thursday workouts are going to be different from your Tuesday/Friday workouts. This helps shock the body and makes sure that you're targeting the muscles from all angles. By making the weights lighter and moving into the higher rep range on some days, and using heavier weights with the lower rep range on the other days you will help train your body for both strength and muscular endurance.

Circuit Training Workout

Finally we come to our last type of workout - the circuit style of training. Remember, this is not your typical gym workout where the exercises are timed between stations. Instead, you are alternating between exercises in the chart below.

Instead of doing all the sets for each exercise before moving on to the next exercise, you're going to do the following: Do one set of one exercise, move to the next set of the next, and so on and so forth until you have cycled through the entire group.

Once you've cycled through once, take a short rest period, catch your breath or get a sip of water (highly recommended!) and return for a second round. Ideally, you should aim to complete three rounds. However, if you find that after one round you are so fatigued that you can't continue, don't. You will get to three rounds eventually if you just keep working at it.

The following two workouts should be alternated. Ideally, you should aim to perform three workouts a week. However, if you can only do two you will still see results.

Also, remember to take a full day of rest between these sessions in order to let your muscles recover. Unlike the upper/lower split, you will be hitting each muscle group in each workout so you cannot perform two sessions back to back.

Day One

Exercise	Sets	Reps
Chest Press	3	8-12
Squats	3	8-12
Shoulder Press	3	8-12
Deadlift	3	8-12
Lateral-Pull-Down	3	8-12
Calf Raise	3	8-12
Horizontal Row	3	8-12
Hanging Leg Raise	3	8-12

Day Two

Exercise	Sets	Reps
Incline Press	3	8-12
Step-Ups	3	8-12
Bent Over Row	3	8-12
Deadlift	3	8-12
Leg Extension	3	8-12
Hamstring Curl	3	8-12
Crunch On An Exercise Ball	3	8-12

Now you have a sample of all three workouts. These are going to be extremely effective for helping you burn off body fat, ramp up your metabolism, and create a defined, strong body.

Again, consult YouTube if you're not sure how to do any of the exercises.

SECTION 2: GIVING YOUR DIET A TUNE UP

Now that you finally know how to work out to burn off body fat, build long lean muscles, and rid yourself of countless hours of boring exercise, it's time to switch gears and have a closer look at your diet!

For many women, the diet is just as problematic as the workout. Carbs or no carbs, gluten or no gluten, fat or no fat?? There is WAY too much conflicting information out there. Getting your diet correct is extremely important since correct food intake is WAY more important than exercise in the fat loss game.

It can be incredibly difficult to understand the best approach to dieting since there are so many different programs out there. Unless you have a PhD in Nutrition, the chances of you feeling confused are quite high. From my experience, even some folks WITH a PhD are confused!

Let's break this down into smaller, digestible steps so that you can finally see exactly what you need to do in order to get the best results possible.

CHAPTER 11: SET CALORIE LEVELS CORRECTLY

What's the one thing that will make or break your efforts with fat loss? Is it avoiding carbohydrates completely? Is it not eating anything past 7 PM? Or perhaps the real ticket to stripping that fat from your body is avoiding food during the few hours after your workout so that your body keeps using all that fat as fuel?

If you answered yes to any of those, you are WRONG.

The single factor that will determine whether or not you lose body fat (or muscle mass, for that matter) is how many calories you take in on a week-by-week basis.

Make no mistake about it, there's no way to overcome eating too many calories. It's pure physics. You must take in less energy than you burn in order for your body to use fat as fuel. If your body is getting plenty of energy each day to meet its needs, why would it ever want to *break down* body tissue (ie. body fat)?

We want to accomplish fuel burning in the most efficient way possible. Fortunately, breaking down body tissue for fuel is just not that efficient. Your body will favor the calories coming in before turning to stored energy.

So before you get yourself all worked up over your carb, fat, or protein intake, you must set calories. There's no other place to start a diet. Let's take a moment to get this straight once and for all.

The amount of calories that you require on a daily basis is broken down into three different components. First, you have your basal metabolic rate (BMR). This stands for how many calories it would take your body to maintain life if you did nothing but lay in bed all day long.

You didn't get up and walk around the house, you didn't eat lunch, and you didn't even read a book – you lied there and slept. That represents your basal metabolic rate.

For most women, you can estimate the basal metabolic rate fairly accurately by multiplying your body weight by a factor of ten.

So if you weigh 140 lbs your BMR is 1400 calories.

One thing to note is this method can be somewhat flawed for women who are either very over fat or very muscular. Fat requires very few calories on a daily basis to exist, while muscle requires many. Therefore, when you have someone at either end of the spectrum, the BMR estimation is flawed.

Those who have more fat mass should adjust their BMR result lower while those who have more muscle mass should adjust higher. Adjust the number you get from the equation by 10% either way and see how you do.

Remember that these are just estimation methods and are not set in stone. One thing to always keep in the back of your mind is that you will have to adjust your calorie intake as time progresses based on the results you see.

Okay, so now that you have that BMR number, it's time to move on to the second factor that goes into determining how many calories to eat.

This factor is referred to as the Thermic Effect of Food (TEF). This factor represents how many calories your body is going to burn by digesting the food you eat. Whenever you eat a meal your body is going to start burning up calories to get that food broken down into usable components.

This is one area where you can actually give yourself a nice metabolic boost simply by eating more protein, which we'll go into later. For now, a good approximate estimation of this will be about 10% of your basal metabolic intake. So for example, if you weigh 140 lbs, your BMR is 1400, and your TEF is (1400*10%)=140.

Moving on, we come to the third and final component of figuring out how many calories you will burn each day and that is the activity factor. This factor is what will vary widely based on how much you're moving in the day. If you sit in your desk all day and hardly move a muscle, your activity factor will be almost zilch.

On the other hand, if you're up running errands, chasing that train before it leaves 3x a day, or have a very active job that keeps you moving plus you're doing regular workouts on top of this, then your activity factor will be far more significant.

What you're going to do now is use a multiplication factor. Take the sum of BMR and TEF and multiply it by:

1.2 if you sit around all day

1.3 if you have a somewhat active job

1.4 if you are following all the workouts that we discussed above

1.5 if you have an active job and are doing your workouts

1.6-2.0 if you're essentially superwoman and never sit down during the day

This is how many calories you require to *maintain* your body weight.

You don't want to maintain your body weight, do you? If you

want to get that lean, defined physique, you need to take in fewer calories than you burn.

You may be tempted to decrease your intake by 1000 calories a day (if some is good, more is better, right?). Don't be so quick to do this. Remember, the body has a very strong protective instinct and when it senses that calories are way too low; it's going to fight back – and fight back *hard*. After all, our ancestors needed to conserve energy (ie calories) in a famine!

The longer you set your calories very low, the more you risk your metabolism severely slowing down. This will result in a plateau. Not to mention, the minute you increase your calories you will gain weight!

Slow and steady, as much as you may hate it, is what will win the race. I recommend shooting for somewhere between 1/2 and 1 pound of total fat loss each week. Those who are more overweight can shoot for 2 pounds per week, at maximum. If you go past this, it's likely to be muscle mass you're losing and not fat (bad!)

To lose 1/2 pound a week you need to create a calorie deficit of about 250 calories per day. To lose 1 full pound a week, you need a deficit of 500 calories per day. In order to lose one pound of body fat you must create a total deficit of 3500 calories.

Those who are aiming for two pounds a week will require a deficit of 1000 calories, so you really need to be careful. You should never take in fewer than roughly 1200 calories per day in order to ensure good nutrition, so only attempt this large of a deficit if you have a *maintenance* calorie intake of 2200 or greater.

Note that you can also bump up the calorie burn by adding more exercise beyond what you factored into your maintenance equation (above). However, keep in mind that proper balance is key.

Now you can subtract your additional calorie deficit from your daily caloric intake and come to your target fat loss requirement. Note that if you're part of the 0.01% of us that are not aiming for fat loss, just reverse this process and add calories to your maintenance level.

Since women build muscle mass at a very slow pace (especially when compared to men), you will not require very many calories above maintenance in order to gain. Expect one pound or so of muscle per month. All you need to add is 200 calories to your maintenance level.

Chances are that your metabolic rate will speed up slightly when you increase calorie intake, which is why 200 is a good number to go with. Don't think that you can overload yourself and go with 500 extra calories in order to build muscle faster because that's just a fast-track way to add more body fat.

In females there is a distinct limit to how much muscle can be built per week, so taking in more calories than needed will not lead to favorable results.

There you have it – your ideal calorie level. As we mentioned earlier, be sure to monitor this based on the progress you're seeing. If you find you aren't losing weight fast enough, lower your calorie intake. If you're losing weight too fast and are worried you're also losing muscle mass, increase.

This constant adjustment process is what will make sure that you reach your goals, and is therefore a necessity.

CHAPTER 12: THE POWER OF PROTEIN

Now that you've figured out your daily caloric requirements, the next step is figuring out your protein intake. Protein is quite possibly the single most important macronutrient to take in if you want to see results from your diet.

The benefits of getting enough protein are endless. Let's go over just a few to show you just how important this nutrient is.

Hunger Control

The first (and probably most important) benefit you'll see with a higher protein intake is better control of your hunger. The reason for this is that protein has very little impact on insulin levels. Insulin levels drive hunger in the body, so when they are lower you will have no problem sticking to your diet.

One of the biggest benefits of the low carb diets is actually hunger control. You will find that with a meal that contains mostly protein along with some vegetables and some healthy fats you won't be hungry for hours. Conversely, a meal that is mostly carbohydrates will have you back in the kitchen within an hour looking for more. So if your boyfriend insists on going out to "boy food" for dinner, get a large piece of the leanest steak you see on the menu accompanied by some fresh vegetables. A sirloin is usually a good option.

If hunger is something that you struggle with on your diet, boosting the protein up is a wise decision.

Lean Muscle Maintenance

Another reason getting enough protein is essential is that you will maintain your muscle mass as you follow a reduced calorie diet. There is a chance that your body may turn to incoming protein as a fuel source throughout the day, especially when the carbohydrates are lower. By having a bit of extra protein in your diet throughout the day, you can make sure that your needs will be met.

This way even if the body turns to protein for fuel, it will still have more than enough of it left over for tissue maintenance and repair.

This is a vital aspect that will keep you looking and feeling great while stripping the fat. Protein intake IS KEY!

Faster Metabolism

One factor of a higher protein diet that you will LOVE is the fact that it promotes a faster metabolism. Protein is the one macronutrient out of the three (protein, carbs, and fats) that uses up the greatest number of calories in the digestion process.

For every one hundred calories of protein you consume, your body will use up about 25 of those to break it down. This means that just by eating more of this nutrient you give yourself a 25% boost in metabolic burn.

With carbohydrates and fat on the other hand, your metabolic boost is only 2 and 5% respectively. Although you should never have a diet that's composed strictly of protein, you will notice by increasing it you have a higher maintenance calorie intake. This makes the process of fat loss that much easier!

Reduced Bloating

While this factor will not have a direct impact on how much fat you lose as you progress with your program, it will influence how you look. Protein rich diets can help reduce the amount of stomach bloat you experience, which helps you look leaner. So if you have a major event to attend on a Saturday night, keep your diet extra high in protein on Friday and Saturday.

Bloating is a real issue and unfortunately one that's hard to get away from. Carbohydrates tend to store water in the body while protein removes it. Therefore, you can tilt the bloat scales in your favor by boosting up protein content.

Steady Energy Levels

The final reason you should be include plenty of protein in your diet is that it helps you be the superwoman that you are throughout the day. Without enough protein you will see huge swings in blood sugar levels, which really wreak havoc on how you feel. One minute you'll be full of energy and ready to take on the world and the next you'll be zonked out on your desk ready for a mid-afternoon nap.

These highs and lows are not fun at all, and by keeping protein as the better part of each meal you will help avoid this. Since protein dramatically slows down the rate that carbohydrates are digested, by having it with each meal you will see a much steadier stream of release, keeping your energy levels constant.

<u>Setting Your Protein Intake</u>

You need to take in somewhere between 1 and 1.5 grams of protein for each pound of body weight. So if you weigh 150 pounds, you should eat 150 to 225 grams of protein each day.

Lean towards the higher end if you're using a larger calorie deficit (500 calories or more). There's no harm in going higher if you are using a smaller calorie deficit if you feel it will help you stick with your diet.

Now lets talk about how protein intake affects calories. Each gram of protein = 4 calories. Let's say you have a woman named Protein Patty, who weighs 150 pounds and has an average diet requirement of 1800 calories. She decides she is going to go with the full 1.5 grams per pound of body weight, making her protein needs 225 grams/day.

We now take the 225 grams and multiply this by 4 (calories per gram) to get 900 calories total. This is how many calories of the 1800 are going to come from protein. I realize this may seem like a lot, but this is because Patty has a deficit in her calorie intake in order to achieve fat loss. Had that deficit not been there, the protein intake would be a much more proportional percentage of her diet since total calories would be higher.

This means Patty has 900 calories to put forth to her carbohydrate and fat sources, which we will discuss next.

We all know that counting calories is a pain in the butt and not always realistic. The good news is that you only need to count them once or twice before habit settles in. For instance, if you are a woman like Patty who needs 225 grams of protein per day and you decide to eat 5 times a day, you simply divide 225 by 5. Now you have 45 grams of protein per meal. So you know that for each meal you should have either 2 scoops of protein powder, 1 large turkey breast (or 1.5 small ones), etc. It will not take you long to learn what the amount of protein you should be eating looks like. Don't feel like you need to be a slave to calorie counting. Give it a week or two and you'll quickly get the hang of it.

<u>Sources of Protein</u>

Before leaving the topic of protein, let's talk sources. The best sources of protein to consume are those that are going to be almost 100% pure protein. This means chicken breast, turkey, lean red meat, egg whites, fish, seafood, low-fat dairy products, and whey protein powder.

If you want to get more exotic with your protein sources you can look into buffalo, ostrich, and duck.

Now let's shift our focus and help you understand more about carbohydrates and how they are going to factor into your diet for weight loss.

CHAPTER 13: USING CARBOHYDRATES CORRECTLY

L et's talk about everyone's favorite topic – carbs. If you're like most women, you have a love-hate relationship with this food group. You *love* to eat them but *hate* the impact it has on your body.

Remember the Atkins craze? If any of you have ever tried it, you may have noticed that it worked! You DID slim down rather quickly. So what's the problem?

It's important for you to understand the role carbohydrates play in the body as well as in the progress you make. Let's look at a few factors to get a better understanding.

Carbohydrates and Energy Levels

The very first thing to know about carbs is that they keep you functioning and happy. If you've ever tried a low carb diet, it's likely that you've experienced some negative effects. Within about 2-3 days of starting the diet (that's the amount of time it takes for your stored supply of carbs to run out), you were faced with extreme fatigue levels that made you want to call in sick and stay curled up in bed all day long. That's not to say days like this don't happen when you are NOT dieting, but with a very low carb diet the fatigue goes to a whole new level.

The reason for this is because the body senses low fuel intake and is responds. With carbohydrates cut back dramatically, there is nowhere to turn to for energy. In time the body begins to go to fat sources for fuel, but this takes a few weeks.

It may seem like this is ideal for fat loss – you're using up your body fat stores for fuel. However, if you are so low on energy that you can hardly move, chances are you won't be working out. Who wants to feel like crap all the time anyway??

So right off the bat that's one strike against very low carb diets.

Carbohydrates and Metabolic Rates

Another very important thing for you to realize about low carb diets is the impact they have on your metabolism. Out of all three macronutrients (carbs, protein, and fat), carbohydrates contain the most hormones that help regulate your thyroid gland and metabolic rate.

If you stick with a very low carb diet for an extended period of time, these hormones start shifting. Before long you will experience intense cravings for food, you will feel hungry immediately after eating a meal, and you will have even lower energy levels than before. In other words, extreme low carb diets will not make for a very active social life! What's the point of looking hot if no one will see you??

The reason all of these side effects occur is a hormone called 'Leptin', which is the 'body fat monitoring hormone'. It watches how much body fat you have and how many calories you're eating on a daily basis. Whenever either of these starts shifting downwards, it speaks up.

Basically, this hormone is the starvation protector. When it senses big changes happening which could lead to starvation, it starts making the body physiologically want to eat. While initially you may have had an odd food craving here and there, now you're fighting a number of factors that make it next to impossible to stick with your diet. Trust me ladies, even the most strong willed will cave with this amount of hunger. Not worth it.

So again, this is another strike for very low carbohydrate diets. If you include some carbohydrates in your plan (to the amount of at least 100 grams per day), you'll find the Leptin hormone stays at the level that it should.

Carbohydrates and Muscle Mass Loss

Finally, the last point I want to touch on with regards to carbohydrates is the impact they have on lean muscle mass.

When you are attempting to perform intense exercise and there are no carbohydrates available for energy, your body attempts to find another available fuel source. Unfortunately with intense exercise, the body cannot physiologically use fat as a fuel source.

It can't and it won't. Fat cannot be broken down quickly enough to derive enough energy for this type of activity.

Therefore, you need another fuel source. And where does your body turn? That's right – your lean muscle mass.

So once again, this very low carb diet causes you to lose muscle mass, which in turn slows down your metabolism!

As your metabolism plummets further, you experience an even slower rate of fat loss. In some cases you may actually start gaining back body fat since you now have such a low daily maintenance calorie requirement.

Whichever way you slice it, very low carb diets and intense exercise do not go hand in hand. These diets should be avoided at all costs. Fortunately this is good news since I'm almost certain that you'd rather eat carbs!

With the way of training and dieting that I'm illustrating to you in this book, you can do exactly that. It's time to break the fear of carbohydrates that so many women have and get them back in your diet the right way.

Now let's look at the approach you should take to adding carbohydrates to your diet.

<u>The 'Good' Carbs-'Bad' Carbs Story</u>

While some people are still firmly rooted in the belief that there are no 'bad' foods as long as they are all natural, the truth is that if weight loss is your main concern there are certain carbs that should be left for cheat days.

By focusing on the superior forms of carbohydrates you will keep your blood sugar levels under control and prevent fat gain.

The carbohydrates you need to focus on are slower digesting, complex, and naturally occurring. Some examples are: unsweetened oatmeal, brown rice, sweet potatoes (which are slower releasing in comparison to white potatoes), fruits, and vegetables. If you want to eat bread, keep it to a minimum and choose the "sprouted grain" variety.

If you focus your diet strictly around these sources, you're off to a good start. These foods will offer you the most fiber and will help you stay fuller for a longer period of time. This improves the chances that you maintain your desired calorie intake for the day.

A big problem occurs when you turn to overly processed foods for your carbohydrate source. These foods cause you to crave more and more carbohydrates, making it very difficult to stick to the plan.

A simple guideline that I recommend you follow when choosing your carbohydrate sources is to look at how many ingredients the particular food contains. If it's a single ingredient (brown rice, an apple, a carrot, etc), then it's fine to add to your diet.

If the food has an ingredient list longer than your daily 'to-do' list, it's better to skip it.

The only time in the day when you should consume simpler forms of carbohydrates is immediately after your workout. During this time your muscles are hungry for a quick source of glucose to suck right up into the tissue in order to use it for the muscle repair process.

<u>Distribute Your Carbohydrates Through The Day</u>

After you have figured out *what* carbohydrates you should eat, the next step is to figure out *when* to eat them. This will make a difference in not only how you look but also in how you feel.

For the most part you want to consume your most 'starchy' (oats, brown rice, potatoes) carbohydrates earlier in the day, as well as after your workout. This is when your body needs fuel most.

Later in the day you will focus on the slower digesting, lower calorie forms of carbohydrates – your vegetables. These will hardly add any calories to your daily total so you can be liberal.

The only three vegetables that you need to be careful with are peas, potatoes, and squash since they are slightly higher in starch and sugar. Limited amounts are fine, but don't overdo it or the calories will add up.

Fruit is the last type of carbohydrate to discuss. Similar to starchy carbohydrates, you're better off adding them earlier in the day when you are more active. One thing that is important to note is that fruit is actually not the best of choices before and after your workout.

The primary reason for this is because fruit is composed up of two forms of sugars (glucose and fructose –which are the fancy names for the type of sugar molecule). Glucose is the type of sugar that will get into the muscle cells and provide fuel for your workouts. It's the good sugar you want. Fructose, on the other hand, is handled differently and will go to the liver instead. This means that fruit will not help you recover from your workout as well as other foods.

In addition, the body has a limited storage capacity for fructose-rich foods, so if you overdo it you will gain fat.

Fruit provides only a few grams of fructose, which is not something to be concerned over. However, other high fructose foods (anything with high-fructose corn syrup) must be eliminated.

If you limit yourself to one to two pieces of fruit a day as part of your overall carbohydrate intake, you should be fine. The nice thing about fruit is that for many people it helps satisfy the craving for something sweet and makes the dieting process much easier.

<u>Calculating Your Daily Carbohydrate Intake</u>

Finally, we are ready to calculate our daily carbohydrate intake. Since you already know how many calories you should be eating in order to lose weight and you know your optimal protein intake, you can work backwards to determine carbohydrate intake.

Carbohydrates and healthy dietary fat (which we'll talk about in a minute) are both flexible in your diet since they can be adjusted based on your own personal preference. Some people prefer having a bit more fat content in their diet, while others prefer to keep carbohydrates on the higher side.

It's important to determine your own personal preference and adjust your diet accordingly.

For right now, let's assume you are going to have a relatively even split between your fat and carbohydrate intake.

Let's back to our example of Protein Patty. She has a daily calorie intake of 1800 calories and is consuming 225 grams of protein each day (900 calories). She has 900 calories left over to plan out the rest of her diet.

Since we are aiming for an equal amount of protein and carbohydrates, we can add in about 450 calories worth of each nutrient. Since there are four calories per gram of carbohydrate, we have about 112.5 grams (just round up to 115 or down to 110 for convenience sake) per day. Remember, over time this will get very easy to eyeball so you won't have to be as focused on the exact numbers. For example, 25 grams of carbohydrates (or approximately 100 calories worth) would be about a large handful of rice or pasta, one slice of whole grain bread, a small whole grain wrap, or about half a bowl of whole grain cereal. If you initially measure out the serving sizes for a day or two, you should have no problem eyeballing.

Once Patty's carbohydrate intake is set, she can spread it out between each of her meals. Remember, carbohydrates are not like protein in the sense that you don't need to have an equal amount at each meal. You should have a much higher number of grams before and after your workout.

If you work out in the evening you don't want to skimp on carbs post-workout. This may mean eating them closer to bedtime. To adhere to your prescribed daily carb grams, just decrease your intake during the earlier meals of the day. You essentially want to be doing the opposite of what someone exercising earlier in the day would do.

This covers your carbohydrate intake. If you eat the right sources in the correct proportions, carbohydrates will not cause you to gain body fat or make it any harder to lose weight.

The fact that carbs make you fat is a huge myth that far too many people are falling for. Big ups to Dr. Atkins! People found that when they cut out their carbohydrates they immediately began losing weight. This isn't surprising since a reduction in carbs will likely result in a reduction of calories.

Next we're going to look at the last major diet macronutrient, dietary fat.

CHAPTER 14: FABULOUS FATS – THEY ARE NOT TO BE FORGOTTEN

Back in the day fats were a greater enemy than carbohydrates. Everyone was turning to very low-fat diets and 'fat-free' snack foods. Manufacturers were using any method they could to provide consumers with reduced fat foods to fit their weight loss diets.

What these dieters failed to realize is that when they cut the fat, they often added extra sugar to the food (or in some cases a sugar replacement which causes numerous gastrointestinal problems).

Now that the low-carb era is upon us everyone is looking for low-carb foods and favoring dietary fat.

While neither approach is entirely correct, there is no reason to completely avoid dietary fat. However, you need to make sure that you're choosing your sources wisely.

Here is some background info about dietary fat and how it relates to weight loss.

Calories In Fat

The first thing you need to keep in mind about dietary fat is the number of calories it contains. Unlike protein and carbohydrates, fat has 9 calories per gram.

This means you can't eat as much fat as carbs and protein. Imagine one tablespoon of olive oil next to one cup of bran cereal. Both have about the same number of total calories, but the cereal obviously has more volume.

Fat takes up much less room on your plate so it can be easy to overeat. If you choose to have a cup of nuts, for example, expect to take in five hundred calories. Obviously this makes weight loss difficult, so it's very important to take the time to measure out your serving sizes.

Fats and Hunger

The second thing to know about dietary fat is the impact they have on hunger. While fat takes up less room on the plate, it tends to be highly satisfying. While carbohydrates spark hunger, fats blunt it. One trick to help reduce the amount you eat is to have a very small amount of nuts about an hour before the meal.

Fat And Energy

The next point to discuss with regards to fat intake is the impact it has on energy levels. As we discussed in the carbohydrate section, fat itself cannot be used as a fuel source when you are doing highly intense exercise. The body cannot convert fat to fuel quickly enough.

Instead, fat can be used as a long-term energy source. The body turns to glucose first (carbohydrates) if it is available. If all carbohydrates have been used up, the body turns to fat energy. This makes sense if you think about it since the body stores fat tissue for times of starvation.

Types Of Fats

Now that you see the benefits of fat, it's time to talk about the sources. Trans fats, which are a mechanically altered type of fat, are the main ones to avoid. In fact, if you can completely eliminate this form of fat from your diet. You will be better off.

Our body has absolutely no need for trans fats. Trans fats are most commonly found in 'shelf' products. This fat is added to food to help shelf life, as well as add taste. Since common sense tells you that these foods shouldn't be part of an overall healthy diet anyway, eliminate them.

The good types of fats that you want to consume are unsaturated and polyunsaturated fats. These will promote healthy cholesterol levels and help support a number of essential body functions. Women who don't consume enough of these fats may begin to see their menstrual cycle stop (particularly when calories are low), so it's vital that you're taking them in.

The best sources of these fats include olive oil, nuts, nut butters, seeds, fatty fish, safflower oil, sesame oil, sunflower oil, and avocados. Getting a good mixture of these in your regular diet is ideal.

Saturated fat has gotten a very bad rap for being highly detrimental to the body. Most people believe that it should be avoided completely. However, smaller amounts of saturated fat are ok since it is often found in foods that you should be eating for other nutrients (cottage cheese and lean steak for example). As long as you can keep it to about 15% of your total fat intake, you're doing fine.

Finally you have essential fatty acids. These are an absolute must for proper health. Essential fatty acids are found in foods such as salmon, mackerel, flax seeds, flax seed oil, walnuts, and sardines.

How Much Fat To Eat

Finally, we have to assess how much fat you should be consuming for optimal results. Generally speaking, you should never go below 15% of your total calories. In some cases you can even bring overall fat intake up to 30-35% depending on how the rest of your diet is laid out. Since your protein intake stays constant regardless, bringing the fat intake up just means carbohydrates must come down. Remember, you have a limited number of calories you can eat each day.

Now, let's look back on our example of Protein Patty. She has a calorie intake of 1800 calories. 900 calories (or 225 grams) are coming from protein rich foods, 450 calories (or 115 or so grams) are coming from carbohydrates, which leaves another 450 calories to come from fat sources. Since there are nine calories per gram of fat, she gets a total of 50 grams of fat per day.

This fat should be spread out over the course of the day, but left out from the meals before and right after the workout period. During these times fat will slow the delivery of nutrients to the muscle tissue, which is not what you're going for.

Generally speaking, meals that are higher in carbohydrates are lower in fat, and vice versa.

Now that Patty has her full diet plan, her next step is to divide it up into meals and place in foods that will meet her requirements. Don't stress if you don't hit your exact targets at the end of each day. As long as you're within a range on a continual basis, you're good. Some days you may be slightly higher in fat while other days you're higher in carbohydrates, and that's fine as long as you don't go to extremes

Now that we have all the main nutrients set out, let's have a look at what Patty's sample meal plan would look like.

Breakfast: 1 whole egg + 2 egg whites scrambled up with your choice of chopped veggies. 1 cup of oatmeal with one tablespoon of peanut butter stirred in.

Mid-Morning Snack: 1 cup low sugar yogurt with ½ scoop of protein powder stirred in with ½ cup fresh berries. Quick and easy.

Lunch: 4 oz grilled chicken breast with two cups of mixed greens and one tablespoon of olive oil based salad dressing. Eat an apple afterwards for a sweet treat.

Mid-Afternoon Snack: One can of light tuna and ¼ cup salsa with one small whole grain wrap. Have one cup of carrot sticks and celery on the side to help boost fiber intake.

Dinner: 5 oz Tilapia with ½ cup of brown rice and 2 cups of steamed vegetables drizzled with one tablespoon of olive oil.

Before Bed Snack: ½ cup of cottage cheese with 1 tbsp natural peanut butter stirred in.

This wraps up our discussion on diet. Getting your diet sorted out will have an incredibly large impact on the results you see. While it is a lot of work, it is well worth the effort. You'll also likely find that after a while tracking your calories will come more naturally and you won't have to be so rigid any longer. You'll just 'know' what to eat and how much is enough.

If you find fat loss start to stall, just start track again just to be sure you are really within your calorie and macronutrient range. Many people who don't track calories or serving sizes will grossly overestimate how much they are eating. By starting off tracking and counting you won't fall into the habit of misjudging what you're eating.

CHAPTER 15: SMART SUPPLEMENTS FOR GETTING SLIMMER

After you have your diet in check, you may want to start looking into some supplements that can help you take things to the next level.

Don't get me wrong, I'm not one to go and promote all those fancy fat burners or overly hyped products you see gracing the latest pages of Shape magazine. There is way too much money being spent in the supplement industry on a variety of products that completely fail to deliver.

The more you get caught up in the all the hype, the lower your chances of success are. You'll be so focused on the latest and greatest product that you'll forget about the tried and true basics – good nutrition and a solid workout plan.

Let's have a very brief look at some of those 'hype' supplements that you should avoid.

Fat and Carb Blockers

The first supplement that you should avoid is anything that states it will block certain nutrients from being absorbed into the body. The problem with these 'blockers' is that they can stop certain essential nutrients from being absorbed as well, which could really put your long-term health in jeopardy.

If you think that by taking these 'magical' supplements you will be able to eat all the carbs or fat that you want and not have any repercussions, you are sorely mistaken.

Fat Burners

The next group of supplements that you should avoid is fat burners. While these may contain ingredients that help you fat loss, they will not replace a bad diet.

Too many people get stuck thinking that just by taking the supplement they will lose body fat.

They will help very slightly. Usually this is done by enhancing energy levels or by blunting hunger. However, the damage these supplements do to your body far outweighs the benefits.

Who wants to walk around in a state of anxiety all day?? This definitely can't be good for you

Now, let's have a peek at the supplements that can make your life just a little bit easier.

Whey Protein Powder

The first supplement that is worth investing in is a quality whey protein powder. If you're like most women, getting in all that protein is quite tricky because you don't especially like feasting on chicken breasts or egg whites all day.

To help make life easier, supplement with protein powder. It's quick, convenient, and if you shop around for a good brand it actually don't taste all that horrible. What's nice is that you can add your protein powder to a number of foods such as oatmeal, cottage cheese, or a shake. This makes it relatively easy to meet your protein requirements. If you're confused about what brand to buy, an excellent choice is Jay Robb Whey Protein Powder due to its lack of extra artificial ingredients.

Remember, failing to meet your protein needs is one of the biggest mistakes you could make in your fat loss diet, so be sure you get enough in.

Caffeine

Moving on, the next supplement to consider is caffeine. You may already be best friends with your morning latte, so you'll be happy to hear that some caffeine immediately before your workout can give you a quick energy burst and help the body utilize fat at an accelerated rate.

If you're not into drinking a full cup of coffee before hitting the gym, consider downing a shot of espresso instead. It will make for less fluid swishing around in your stomach while you're jumping around.

If you choose to use caffeine, make sure that you don't overdo it or you could find yourself having problems sleeping or becoming dependent. 200 mg per day is more than enough.

Fish Oil

The third supplement that I highly recommend is fish oil. Unless you're consuming a high amount of flax seeds and fatty fish each week, using this supplement will make it easier to meet your essential fatty acids requirement.

Take 2-4 caps divided into two doses throughout the day. Try Carlson Laboratories - Very Finest Fish Oil. It is one of the best quality fish oils available on the market.

If you're eating correctly and following a proper workout program, you won't have much of a need for any type of supplement. Make these your lowest priority.

SECTION 3: MAINTAINING YOUR PROGRESS – BEAT THAT PLATEAU

Finally, the last section of this book deals with something that is very near and dear to almost every woman out there – the dreaded plateau. All of a sudden, you work out and eat clean and NOTHING HAPPENS! Chances are you've experienced this at some point and possibly even quit your program as a result.

The program presented here is going to be very different since you won't plateau nearly as often. As long as you follow the guidelines I have given you, results will continue for a long period of time.

However, it is inevitable that at some point progress will slow down. This is a normal occurrence and happens to everyone. You must be prepared with some tools in your arsenal to fight back and get you on the road to results.

Let's take a look at some of the major issues you might encounter and exactly what you are going to do to get past them.

CHAPTER 16: MONITORING YOUR PROGRESS

L adies, why do we bust our ass? RESULTS!

Before we talk about what to do to break through your plateau, let's take a look at what you must do to monitor your progress. Seeing progress is THE BEST motivator out there.

The most popular method of measuring results is weighing yourself on the scale. If you are like most women on a fat loss quest, you begin each day by steppig on the scale.

While this is a helpful tool for determining your weight, it does very little in telling you how well your program is working. Remember our discussion of muscle vs fat? Unless you know you are losing *body fat* you really don't know much about your progress at all.

In fact, you may see the scale go down while you are actually moving backwards from your goal. Hard to imagine, but true. This is why the "Skinny Jeans" method is a much wiser option.

The Skinny Jeans Method

It is very difficult to see physical changes in your body since you look at yourself in the mirror every day. Have you ever lost weight and only noticed because someone else told you? Gradual changes are extremely hard to see. This is why it is easier to see a *relative* change. Relative to a pair of jeans, that is. Choose a pair of jeans that are slightly tight on you, and as time goes on watch them get looser! Perhaps your sides will hang over less, or perhaps your tummy will look tighter. The type of change will depend on your body type, but one sure thing is that there will definitely be a change if you follow the advice in this book.

If you are ambitious, the body fat test method is also an effective way to monitor progress.

The body fat test will indicate to you how much of your weight loss has been fat (good) and how much has been muscle (bad). In some cases you may find that your fat has gone down while the muscle and body weight has gone up, which indicates progress.

So how do you get a body fat test done? There are a few different options.

Skin Calipers

The first method of testing your body fat is with skin calipers. A personal trainer in a gym usually does this. In this method the skin caliper will pinch an area of skin and determine the thickness of that pinch (which represents body fat).

This is done in a few different regions on the body and then the readings are plugged into an equation. This gives you a rough estimate of how much body fat you have.

The drawback to this approach is that it tends to be somewhat inaccurate since you also contain a lot of body fat within the organs and internal structures of the body. It's also a bit of a pain in the butt to constantly have to find someone to pinch your fat.

Hand-Held Devices/Scales

Another method of testing body fat is hand held devices (or sometimes a scale that you step on similar to your standard scale). This works by sending an electrical current through the body, which assesses the conductivity of the tissues.

If the current passes very quickly, you have more muscle mass and less body fat. If it passes slowly you have a greater overall percentage of fat mass.

The pros to the hand-held device approach are that it is cheap and quick to do. The main con of these devices is that the measurement can be extremely swayed by small factors, such as whether you had a glass of water prior to the test. If you want to give this a shot a good choice would be the Omron Fat Loss Monitor. If you take your body fat at the same time every morning before ingesting any food or water you will get a reasonably good indicator of your progress.

This wraps up the discussion of the various methods used to assess body fat. It is very important that you find a way to determine your progress that isn't related to the scale so that you have an accurate picture of progress.

The Progress Journal – Your Ticket To Success

Next we come to another key element for making sure you can beat a plateau and stay motivated – the progress journal. This allows you to look back over time and make sure that you are seeing results.

How many times have you had a problem in your life that you thought you had NO IDEA how to deal with until you talked out loud to a girlfriend about it or wrote it down in a journal? Working out and getting in shape is very similar – although it's a pain in the butt to write everything down, until you do I PROMISE you will not keep nearly as good track of your progress. Without a journal it will be much more difficult to figure out what you need to tweak. Therefore, no journal = slower results.

Another huge added benefit of having a progress journal is that when you are having a bad day and feel like nothing you do is making a difference, you can look back see just how far you've come. Very often we forget where we started and only focus on the day to day, which can really push things out of perspective.

Luckily, in this day in age there are some excellent online tools to help you monitor your progress. My favorite site is The Daily Burn. And don't worry, there's an app for that so you can use it on your phone. Remember, it is normal to see weight loss slow down as you get closer to your goal weight so don't expect to see the same results the whole time. This slow down is natural since the less extra body fat you have, the more the body will hold on to your existing fat mass.

By keeping track of your progress in a journal you'll be able to see the small changes taking place and give yourself the reassurance that what you are doing is working.

So what do you write in your progress journal?

Ideally, you want to write down the amount of weight you're using for each exercise, how many reps and sets you perform, and how you feel. This feeling aspect is important because it allows you to see when you are in need of a good break from your training. This can be easily tracked in The Daily Burn.

If at any point you find that getting those workouts in is becoming something you dread because you're so tired all the time, you need to seriously consider some time off. The body can only handle so much exercise for any given period before starts to struggle to recover. By consistently watching for this lack of energy you will stop fatigue before it becomes unmanageable.

If you're up for it, write down what you eat. Again, easily taken care of in The Daily Burn. This tremendously helps your accountability.

So get started on a journal immediately when you begin your new program. After a week or two of regular entries, it will be a natural part of your day and you may even find that you really look forward to it.

CHAPTER 18: ANTICIPATE OBSTACLES

Things happen. Your girlfriends plan a trip to Vegas, you have one too many drinks on Saturday night and end up eating a large burrito, or you get the flu. This is life. It is IMPERATIVE that once the obstacle is over (whether it be 2 days or 2 weeks) you get back on track. I cannot tell you how many times these things have happened to me and I wanted to say screw it all! Don't do it. Jump back on track.

Remember, a small setback is just that: *a small setback.* There's no reason to let this become a big setback and get off track completely.

One bad meal is easy to undo. A week of bad eating is not so easy. You get the point. Don't let one tiny slip-up lead to disaster.

When a setback does occur, it helps to be prepared. Here are some ways you can do that.

1. Come Up With A Shortened Workout Solution

If it's time that's creating the barrier, try and figure out some shorter workout solutions. Let's say you can't get into the gym for your regular hour-long session. This does not mean you need to skip it entirely.

Instead, just go to the gym and perform one set of each exercise that you would typically do. This single set is still going to invoke a muscular response and will get you closer to your goals.

Or, stay home and hit the TRX.

2. You're Stuck Without Food And Your Stomach Is Rumbling

Your best bet is to always be prepared. Stash something in your purse, car, or at the desk in the office.

Examples here would be protein powder, a tin of pop-top tuna, a small bag of nuts, or a homemade protein bar.

These snacks are just 'there' for you – *always*. They are the snacks that you turn to when you aren't prepared with a real snack and are attempting to avoid the vending machine.

If you aren't prepared, then you simply make the most of it. Always try and find a snack that has the most protein since that's what will help you stay on track and help stop hunger pangs. The worst thing you could do is go for a very low protein, high simple carb snack since it will not fill you up.

Bad idea.

One final note is that there is no shame in just not eating. If you can manage and you're not totally famished, just don't eat. Wait till you can get to a healthy option. I promise that being a few hours late for your regularly scheduled meal will not put your body in fat storage mode.

3. You Had Too Much To Drink

Drinking too much often leads to indulging in foods that were *not* on the plan.

When this happens, your best bet is to just rest one day and get back on the plan. One day of too much alcohol and calories isn't going to set you back to square one. It may hinder progress slightly, but this can easily be fixed with two or three solid days back on.

The most important thing is that you don't dwell on it and lose all your motivation.

Instead, use your setback as a motivational tool – get upset that you went off track, but use that feeling to push harder in your workouts during the coming week.

Keep these tips in mind. Setbacks will happen; it's part of life. How you handle these setbacks is what determines whether you influence your *long-term results.*

CHAPTER 19: METHODS TO PUSH PAST A PLATEAU

One key thing to remember about results is NO PAIN NO GAIN. You should feel very challenged when you work out. If something feels easy or moderate, it's time to switch it up.

Although breaking past a plateau is a lot simpler than you think, many women have a hard time doing it mentally. After 1 week of a certain routine, you will find it EXTREMELY comfortable to come back to the gym and do the same routine. It gets easier and more familiar. Routine is easy, change is hard. Don't let it be so hard, just tweak a few minor things. I guarantee it will go a long way.

Here are some quick ways to overcome a plateau.

Switch Your Exercises

A good way to push past your plateau is to switch your exercises so that your body is exposed to a brand new form of stimulus. For instance, if you've always done back squats, maybe it's time to try some front squats. Or if you've been using dumbbells, try barbells. It seems like you're using the same muscles, but you'll be surprised at how much you have to lower the weight. THIS IS GOOD. It means you are challenging the body in a new way. As a general rule, switch your exercises once a month.

When you do the same thing all the time your body quickly adapts. This is when it begins to sit back and relax. You NEVER want this. By forcing your body to try something new, you're also forcing it to change. This is when results will come.

Add Some Supersets

Another way to shake up the workout is to add some supersets. This means that you perform one set of an exercise and then immediately move on and perform another set of a second exercise without rest.

Once both sets have been completed you can rest and recover before repeating the cycle. The benefit to this is that it increases the intensity of the workout program while also decreasing the total time you're at the gym. Anyone looking to save time will definitely appreciate this approach.

Again, at first this will be hard. This is what you want.

Take A Training Break

Finally, an easy tweak!

In some situations you just need to take time off. If the body isn't recovering properly between workouts, it's not going to matter what you do because you will not see progress.

Some people find that after a week away from their workouts they immediately start seeing results when they get back on it. So if all else fails, consider taking a break.

Reduce Your Rest Periods

As time progresses, one mistake many people make is letting their rest periods go too long. What starts out as a 30 second break slowly drags on to a full minute. Before long, your scheduled 1 minute rests have turned into a chat/flirt session with the hot guy in the weight room. Don't do it. Keep tabs on how much time you take. If you allow yourself to rest for too long you will severely decrease the overall intensity of your workout program and negatively impact your metabolic boost.

For better results, keep the breaks snappy. Attempt to make them even shorter than you normally do (but still make sure you're recovered enough to lift an appropriate amount of weight). This will really make sure that you are working hard.

If you still find yourself stuck in a plateau you should also take a good, hard look at your diet. Again, this is where the journal comes in handy! It could be a matter of consuming too many calories. Always remember that regardless of what you're doing in the gym, if you don't have your eating correct you will see very minimal results.

CHAPTER 20: CONCLUSION

Are you convinced yet? I hope that after taking the time to read through this, you're ready to say goodbye to your old cardio-slavery ways and hop on to this new form of training.

It's time that we changed the way women think about their bodies, their workout styles, and their overall approach to wellness and fat loss. All of the methods that I've presented to you here are tried and true by myself personally.

Ask yourself if your current workouts are getting you the results you want? Chances are they aren't. The only thing that's going to change that is by making a serious overhaul and adopting brand new methods of training.

If you don't do something now, how long will you continue with no results? Weeks? Months? *Years?*

Do you really want to be exactly where you are today five years from now?

I know you will be much happier, healthier, and look a hundred times better with your new approach to fitness. There's absolutely no doubt in my mind that you will notice positive changes in your body.

So don't just finish this book and carry on with what you're doing. I urge you to *use* this information. Knowledge only becomes power when it's put into action. Start taking steps right now for long-term results.

www.ingramcontent.com/pod-product-compliance
Lightning Source LLC
Chambersburg PA
CBHW051221250726
48655CB00006B/2532